The All-Food Diet

Hans Guttmann

Please visit the blog and FaceBook page. Feel free to ask any questions, post any thoughts or ideas you may have, or just talk about your health, the things you did (or didn't) do today, food, activity, or whatever interests you.

www.facebook.com/AllFoodDiet

AllFoodDiet.blogspot.com

www.amzn.com/gp/product/148009966X

www.goodreads.com/book/show/16145627-the-all-food-diet

Table of Contents

ACKNOWLEDGMENTS

For Jeanette, the galley slave

Thanks to my literate family members.
I am the least educated of the bunch.

Allen (& Doris)
Betty
Britt
Erika (& Jerry)

Front cover photo by Pat McGrath

HOW THE ALL FOOD DIET CAME ABOUT

I have always been thin. Partly this is genetics, but the other factors are diet and lifestyle. My diet is pretty good, and I lead an active lifestyle. My ex noted one day "when we were together I lost weight". Wow, that was easy. People go through the most extraordinary lengths to lose weight and improve their health. It doesn't have to be that difficult.

What does All-Food mean? First, avoiding chemicals in your food. Secondly, avoiding processed food. The guiding principle is to buy foods with only one ingredient. These are good foods. Foods with many ingredients tend to be bad. Single ingredients good: rice, carrot, lentils, oranges. Many ingredients bad: canned soup, frozen dinners, Doritos.

A clarification. Once you have bought foods with a single ingredient, you are encouraged to combine as many of them as you like in the formation of meals. You can make your own soups, stews, and sauces, but don't buy them pre-made.

For millennia, people searched for the fountain of youth, arduously crisscrossing the known world. They could have used it too, as their life expectancy was about half of ours. Now we know how to live a long healthy life. Don't smoke, sleep, eat right, and exercise. What are people's reaction to this knowledge? They reject health as being too difficult to achieve.

A bit about me for perspective. I'm 6'2", 165 lbs. I live in Minneapolis near the bike path. Do I practice what I preach? No, not all the time. But many of these suggestions come from my own lifestyle.

This book is not an instruction guide that you must follow to the letter. It is composed of a few main ideas, and a host of suggestions. Feel free to take or leave the suggestions. If you follow some of the basic principles, your health should improve, and your quality of life with it.

I talk a lot about losing weight. What I really mean by that is to be healthy, get more muscle tone, feel better, and have more stamina. It's fine to be a little heavy as long as you feel fit. Rather than be long winded about this all the time, I just say 'low fat' or 'lose weight'. Now that we've got our terminology straight, lets talk turkey. Or tofu as the case may be.

There are three main themes in the book, eating well, living an active lifestyle, and being green. Being green is only vaguely connected to the first two themes, but I like the idea. If you can incorporate it into your lifestyle, kudos to you.

There are a lot of diets out there, and a lot of methods for losing weight. Some involve extreme privation, or surgery. Some seem ridiculous at first glance, and for that matter, at second glance. Some involve pills, some deprive you of nutrition. The All-Food Diet is none of that. It consists of simple common sense habits, all of which are optional. Each little thing you do will incrementally improve your health, and become a habit that requires little effort or discipline to maintain.

Disclaimers: I am not a doctor. Be careful biking, as the

instruction manual for my bike intones: Don't bike at night, without a helmet, without a light, during the day, on the street, or on the sidewalk. Use training wheels if you under 21 years of age. When weight lifting, have your team of physicians initial your chart between each rep, certifying that you are healthy enough for the next one.

LET'S TALK ABOUT FOOD

The kitchen is the center of your home, a place to relax, work together, and socialize. Hang out there. Invite friends over. Spending time preparing and consuming food should be a pleasure, not a duty. Socializing is better done in the kitchen than the TV room.

Cook for yourself, your partner, your friends. You don't need to cook just at mealtime. Cook when you are bored, have free time, feel like listening to the radio, or have company over. I cook when I wake up too early. Sunday is a good time to cook for the week, making mass quantities of good food.

Cooking is a good shared activity. One person can chop veggies, or wash dishes while the other prepares the food. What is the point of all this cooking? It's a way to socialize without subjecting yourself to calorie-laden restaurants. Putting the effort into cooking will lead you to healthier meals. Your leftover soup will be more appealing and healthier than any frozen entrée.

How does one make a meal? Some people claim that they don't know how to cook. Perhaps their idea of cooking is opening a can, or microwaving something. Fortunately, our fore-mothers have provided us detailed instructions on food preparations. These are called "Cook books". If you find them intimidating, invite a friend over to help you with the basics. Some people will say 'there is nothing to eat in the house'. What they are really saying is there is nothing that can be ready in five minutes. A few foods and a little creativity can make a fine meal. A little rice, an onion, butter... that's almost enough to make dinner.

Now that you have visualized your inner chef, lets talk about food. We'll break it down into three categories, good food, bad food, and OK food, which is in between.

BAD FOODS

Bad foods have more than one ingredient. They also tend to have fat, salt, sugar, and chemicals. Here are some bad foods:

Canned food is to be avoided. It's fatty, salty, and not necessary. Fresh food is preferable to canned. If something isn't in season, you can buy something else that is. Summer is the time for fresh green veggies. Winter is the time for potatoes, onions, apples, cabbage, and carrots. We're going to give up on the idea that every food is available 365 days year, in exchange for the idea that when a given food is fresh it will taste better. That is, unless you live in a climate like California, in which case the food is fresh year round.

Canned soup is particularly unhealthy. For one thing, it has too much salt. Low-salt varieties also have too much salt. This fact comes from the list of 'ten foods you should never eat'.

Junk food is bad. If you must eat it, I would suggest not keeping any in the house. That way there will be fewer temptations to resist. As you eat more and more real food, you may find that you lose your taste for junk food.

High Fructose Corn Syrup is also to be avoided. Read the label. Look carefully at juice. The words "Drink" and "Cocktail" are giveaways, indicating its presence. Real sugar is better than corn syrup. Better yet is brown sugar, molasses, and honey. You can also skip the sweeteners. For instance, herb tea tastes fine unsweetened, and pancakes are yummy with butter and spreadable fruit.

Accent, which is actually MSG, is a classic example of a non-food. Not having any in your home is easy enough. The trick is to remember to ask that it be omitted in oriental restaurants. If they can't do that, that's not a great sign, and you might consider another restaurant. People lived for centuries and made great food without MSG.

Artificial sweeteners and additives. This includes NutraSweet and all sorts of things. None of them qualify as food. And Olestra? There are side effects. Some of them are unpleasant. Do you want to put these unnatural things into your body? No, you don't. Ever.

Preservatives are bad too. Is this starting to sound complicated? This is why the one ingredient rule works so well. It's easy to remember, and you know that whatever you are buying will be natural.

Fast food is not terribly healthy. I make it a point not to set foot between the golden arches. What would the world be like if everyone did that? A better place. The others fast food joints I visit occasionally. I used to go to Subway, but then found that I could do better by going to the supermarket for lettuce, cheese, and good bread. Also note that fast food uses a lot of disposable packaging, which is quite ungreen. Avoiding fast food will go a long way towards improving your health.

FOOD, DIETS, AND HEALTH

Some people have pretty strange diets. You think they wouldn't work, but sometimes they do. My friend Ivar ate and drank only at dawn. He subsisted on crackers and canned peaches. Later on, he lost weight with a pizza and mountain dew diet. Don't ask me how this works.

Who thinks vitamins make you healthy? Lots of people. That's why Americans have the world's most expensive urine. I suggest taking vitamins sparingly. Natural is better, but watch out for the expensive ones. Are they really any better than the cheapos? I take a multivitamin, and some others as the mood strikes me.

I heard a talk on the radio about diet X. It claimed you'd lose tons of weight, have better skin, and be healthy for taking this supplement. I'm suspicious, and the claims seem exaggerated. We all know that most diets lead to yo-yo weight gains. Worst of all, I think the diet X supplement consisted of chemicals. This is not the road to health.

A lot of people are talking about "no" diets. No Gluten, no wheat, no carbs? All-Food Diet is one thing but this is starting to sound like a No-Food Diet, a flight whose final destination is the grave. If you think you have headaches, skin problems, depression, low energy, or allergies that are caused by these things, try cutting them out and see if it works for you. If you have no problems, feel free to eat bread and grains. Carbs can be good.

If you really want to be healthy, look over the All-Food Diet and note the ideas that you think will blend with your lifestyle. While it's a good idea to get up at six every morning and exercise an hour, most people won't do it regularly. Make a habit of things that make sense to you. It shouldn't be a struggle to be healthy, it should just be part of your daily routine.

Bad habits present a hump you need to get over. Processed food sends your brain several messages. One is "Yum", and another is "More more more". Once you go through withdrawal, you'll be repelled by much processed food, and attracted to natural food.

I let y'all slide on sweets earlier, but they are a good place to start. If you can reduce, not bring home, not order, not sample, cut down, or eliminate sweet things you'll be the better for it. We're talking processed sweets here. Fruits are OK.

Cutting down other places has its benefits as well. Once a week, can you substitute a healthy restaurant for an unhealthy one? Or a meal at home for one out of the home?

While you are at it, try and cut down on heavily fried food too. This is a low hanging fruit, if you can call burgers, fries, or chicken fruit.

Traveling. Out on the open road, you've got problems. There is fast food, and little else. If you are lucky, you'll spot a ma and pa place with real food. More often, they'll feature non-diary creamer, prefab pie, canned veggies, instant or frozen taters, and an excess of salt, fat, and sugar. Your best bet is to bring food, and stop at supermarkets.

Some people have trouble with holiday food. I just don't think excess belongs in a holiday. Halloween is a time to avoid candy. Christmas has nothing to do with spending money, on junk food or anything else. And Easter baskets are a creation of corporations. One Thanksgiving I partook in a 24-hour potato fast. That was my way of reacting to society's over-indulgence. My buddy and I skipped breakfast and dinner, and had a single meal of plain potatoes.

GOOD FOODS

Soupersize it! Soups are underrated. They are a hearty meal that also uses up your leftovers. If you eat meat, it's easy to make a soup with body. If you don't, some trickery is required. What you need is a good base.

Miso works well as a base. You can add things like green onions, baby bok choy, tofu, spicy peppers, and shrimp. I add the Asian rice noodles last. Sometimes I set aside a portion of the soup for today, and add noodles only to it. Otherwise the noodles grow and grow in the fridge, turning the soup into a solid.

Milk makes a good base as well. You can add things like potatoes, onions, celery, clams or fish, and curry powder.

Another trick is to put greens or veggies in the blender. I once blended a giant zucchini and then added veggies to the green liquid. This is a fine way to use up surplus zucchini, lest they procreate and take over the world.

A little oil (not a lot) helps create a base. You can fry onions and other ingredients in olive oil or butter before adding to the soup.

When the soup is done, you can have some, but it'll get better if it sits in the fridge for a day. When it cools, package it in meal-sized portions. If there is too much for the fridge, and you wont be able to eat it in a week, freeze some. Larger frozen portions are good for camping trips, the soup doing double duty as an ice-like cooling agent before metamorphosing into your dinner.

Stock is a good base as well. Save those peelings from potatoes, carrots, broccoli stems, etc. Every so often, take them out of the freezer and boil them a while. Then strain it and keep the broth. You can freeze the stock for later use, or make soup right then and there.

Vegan soups require a little planning. Potatoes and leeks do well together. Blendered cashews can form a base as well.

I happen to like celery, reputed to be a negative calorie food. You can make soup out of celery, potatoes, onions, and milk. Use the leafy part of the celery too. A touch of cumin or curry, some pepper, salt to taste and you are done.

Bread is a staple, also known as the staff of life. The best is your own from scratch. The worst kind is soft, like Wonder bread. The supermarket will have lots of healthy looking breads, but they may contain corn syrup, too many ingredients, and too many chemicals. Bread should be fresh and heavy and dark, with few ingredients. If it's from a local natural bakery eat it quickly, because it will go bad without preservatives. You can also share the loaf, or freeze some. If you can bike to the local bakery, it's a win-win for you.

Stir-fry is another pillar of a healthy eating. Start the brown rice, and then add a few veggies. Three ingredients is enough. For instance, select from onions, baby bok choy, peppers, tomatoes, and tofu. For visual appeal follow the flag rule. Everything you cook should have the colors of the Mexican flag in it. Green, White, and Red. There aren't that many red foods, so plan ahead. It's OK to substitute orange or yellow foods, many of which are quite healthy. Even if your stir-fry comes out bland, avoid fattening it up. Instead, zip it up with hot sauce, curry, and spices.

Dried beans are another staple. Yes, they take a little time to cook. But in return, they last, are inexpensive, and are full of nutrition. Corn and beans make a complete protein, as do rice and beans. Lentils cook quickly, and can be cooked with rice or veggies in the same pot. Dal is a lovely staple to have around all the time. Black beans are good with citrus, pintos in chili, and chickpeas in Indian dishes. Sometimes I pressure cook them, and other times just let them simmer for hours.

Here is a traditional cooking method for pintos and other beans. First look for rocks, pouring out a few beans at a time on a plate and examining them. Then rinse them. Soaking is optional, but if you do soak them, use the soaking water to cook the beans. Add a chopped white onion. Bring to a boil, and simmer on a low heat for hours until they are soft. When they are done, add salt and lime to taste.

It's hard to go wrong with salad. I tend to avoid salad dressing, in favor of a little lemon or lime. A few ingredients will do. Go ahead and add a few calories, in the form of olive oil, avocado, olives, or cheese. Man does not live by lettuce alone.

Fruit is good stuff. Try and eat it every day. I'll blend it into a smoothie, especially if it's imperfect or getting soft. Old bananas make a fine Banana bread.

Pasta is on the good list too. Just say no to pre-made sauce. You can make your own out of olive oil, onions, garlic, tomatoes, peppers, and greens such as broccoli or brussels sprouts.

Hot Cereals tend to be healthy. Grits are tasty, and part of my heritage, but not as nutritious as oatmeal or cream of wheat.

Cold cereal. Try and avoid the usual suspects. They typically have lots of sugar, which is bad, or corn syrup, which is worse. They claim to be filled with vitamins and 'part of a balanced' breakfast, but in reality have little to offer and are expensive to boot. A few, surprisingly, have one ingredient, and I have nothing against them, but I prefer a natural cereal. Look at the box for the fiber number. Aim for 25% or higher. If it tastes like the box, you know it's good for you. Just kidding. Some natural cereals taste fine, just find one that you like.

A note on flour, pasta, rice, and tortillas. Whole-wheat flour is more nutritious than white. Brown rice is superior to white. The same goes for whole-wheat pasta, which has a hearty taste. Try it, you might prefer it. In all these cases, the 'white' product is made by removing the most healthful parts of the food.

Let's talk tofu. People make fun of it. Even if you are a carnivore, you may as well try tofu. Plain it's not very exciting. But it's good fried, where it absorbs some flavours. It also does well in miso soup. Always buy extra-firm. If you are truly terrified to try it at home, try an Asian restaurant. They have loads of tofu dishes, and I guarantee you'll like them.

Spices & Zip. We all want zip with our meals. They shouldn't be bland and boring. The trick is to find ways to add zip without adding fat. Spices and hot sauce are a key here. For stir-fry try pepper, cumin, curry. These work for milk and egg based dishes too. Use hot sauce with everything.

These are not all the good foods out there. That was just a list of some of them, some suggestions in case you had no idea what to do with the pile of real food you just bought. There are more single ingredient foods out there. Bon appetit.

What about the food pyramid you ask? When I was younger, and believed everything I read, I thought that nutritionists and scientists created the four food groups. In fact, the meat and dairy industry gave money to lobbyists who in turn gave it to politicians, and presto, meat and dairy are a food group. And don't get me started on school lunches, which are designed not to be nutritious, but to pay farmers to grow lots of fatty meat and dairy products. The four food groups eventually got replaced by a pyramid, which de-emphasized meat and dairy. But before it could go to press, politicians had their influence, and they toned down the part that pointed you towards healthier food.

OK FOODS

Dairy is OK in moderation. Use it, but not too much. I use real butter. Do you see dairies claiming that their product tastes just like margarine? I use whole milk. You can too. You have my permission. Or you can use 1% or 2% if you prefer. Rice Dream, soy milk and Almond Breeze keep well and are a fine way to cut down on dairy.

Desserts have calories, but I can't put them in the bad list. My readers would rebel. Some people crave desserts, some don't. Making your own has merit, at least you'll know that it will be free of corn syrup and other non-food items.

Chips have little going for them, but I like them. If they have three ingredients (corn, oil, salt) they are OK. If there are more ingredients, that's bad. But wait you say, isn't three more than one? Let me get out my calculator. Yep, it sure is, but I like chips so they get a waiver. Chips are good with hummus and salsa, both of which have more than one ingredient. However, both can be made at home from scratch, something I've done only occasionally. When the chips get old, save them to put in soup. Waste not want not. This works for old bread too.

Pizza isn't the worst food, although it does tend to have calories. Having worked in 11 pizza shops, I'm somewhat tired of it. If you love pizza, go ahead and have it. It doesn't hurt to make it veggie, or to cook your own.

DRINKS

Most people don't drink enough water. Water is good for you, and has zero calories. It's better for you than most drinks. Alcohol, soda, and caffeine all dehydrate you. Try to drink many glasses of water every day. I have a glass of water at my bedside. At work, keep a glass by your desk. Getting up to refill the glass repeatedly gives your eyes a rest from the screen, and stretches the legs a bit. When you are out and about, bring water with you. Seltzer water is also zero calorie, and soothes the stomach. Have all you want.

Juice is good, as long as it's made of food. Look carefully for words on the label like "drink" or "Cocktail", and in the ingredients list for the Corn Syrup. These are to be avoided. Anything that is 100% juice is OK. I find juice to be a little on the strong side, and I often water it down. I call this concoction "juice-water". The glass can be half full (of water). Or it can be 80% full of water. The resulting blend is light and thin, making me want to drink more and more of it. It's zippier than plain water, it's wildly frugal, and it's a way to get more fruit into you.

Herbal tea is great. No calories, no drawbacks. Some teas may even have beneficial properties. Peppermint is reputed to be a panacea.

Green note! Avoid disposable bottles. Bottled water is healthy, but wastes plastic and energy. Most tap water is drinkable. If it's yucky, like in Los Angeles, try an under-sink filter, or have big reusable bottles delivered.

Alcohol is deemed good for you in moderation. Serfs

drank beer every day, as the water was often contaminated. The French love their wine, and they seem healthy enough, it takes two of them to weigh as much as an American. Picture yourself retired on the Riviera with a wineglass in your hand. Wine is fine. That's why Roman slaves were allocated forty-four gallons a year.

Caffeine is not good for me, but it might be OK for you. If you do indulge, try and eat a little something in the morning, and not just have tea or coffee.

HOW MUCH TO EAT AND WHEN TO EAT IT

How much good food should you eat? Generally speaking, as much as you want. I ate copiously as a teen, and kept the habit up for decades, even though it made me uncomfortably full. Now I often use an oversized teacup for my meal portions. Try eating tiny portions, and see if they satisfy you. Your stomach delays a while before sending the full signal to the brain. You can always have more later. You'll be surprised at how little you can eat and be happy about it. Occasionally you'll work hard, play hard, or be out in the cold, and become ravenous. That's the time to eat on the heavier side, not every meal.

And here is a tip for eating less: use chopsticks with every meal. It may slow you down. At my high school, we kept our chopsticks in our mailboxes, making things easier for the silverware washer.

When should you eat? When you are hungry is not a bad answer. Ideally you should eat three meals a day, and not snack much in-between. In particular, try not to eat after dinner.

Eating breakfast is good. I'm not hungry in the morning, but I try to eat something. I usually have high fiber health cereal. Other foods are OK too. I don't keep pastries and the like in the house. Since they aren't around, I don't eat them much.

Dinner should be at a reasonable hour, like 6pm. If it gets to be 8pm or 9pm, skip dinner and wait for breakfast. It won't kill you, and it's better than charging up on calories before bedtime.

WHERE TO BUY FOOD

OK, you say, I understand about this food stuff, how some is good and some is bad. So where do I find real food? Do I have to order it online? You are in luck. Food is widely available. I can walk to four supermarkets, and bike to a dozen or more smaller grocers. At the large grocery stores there is plenty of food. First stroll through the produce area. Then give it a second pass. Then continue looking for real foods, those with one ingredient. Dried beans, bulk food, and some dairy all have their place in your shopping basket.

In some parts of the country it's hard to find things like tofu, hummus, bok choy, coconut milk, rice dream, or sprouts in your local grocer. I once failed to find hummus in a southern market. The cashier had never heard of it. The manager had heard of it, but wasn't sure what it was. I mean, we're talking Middle Eastern staples here, the kind of food that Jesus ate every day. Fortunately this is changing, and supermarkets are expanding their real food section to compete with co-ops and natural food chains.

You will find some good food at a health food chain, such as the one referred to as 'whole paycheck'. If you pick and choose, avoiding prepared foods, the bite will not be so bad. Also, their house brand (365) is reasonably priced. Free samples abound, particularly on Saturday.

Is organic better? Free range? This is a trick question. The definitions of these words keep changing. The answer is maybe. Local is good, chemical free is good, factory farms and GMO are bad. Ultimately, it's up to you. Every time you buy food, you are endorsing certain products with your pocketbook. The people have the power. That's why cod liver oil is no longer a best seller.

Co-ops are great place to find real food, some of which is also local. You can support yours by becoming a member. Mine gives me a small check every year and discounts with every purchase. The co-op is also full of processed health food, which is better than chemical laden processed food, but still should be avoided.

Farmers markets are great too, go as often as you can. Take your bike of course. If you come home with too much food, try and share with others. What do you notice about the food there? It's (hopefully) chemical-free, and contains only one ingredient, the hallmarks of good food.

Trader Joe has some good food items. The produce is good, the house brand is reasonable, and who can go wrong with two-buck chuck?

Asian grocers have lots of great food, and are quite inexpensive. I always try and fill my basket, but sometimes I have to pay cash. There is a $5 minimum for using credit cards, and a full basket only costs four something. This is the kind of problem you want to have. I usually pick up sprouts, limes, baby bok choy, tofu, and upon occasion avocados and assorted Asian noodles. Indian and Middle Eastern grocers are also a fine source of real food.

Convenience stores carry little in the way of food. I avoid them. I also try to avoid low-end supermarkets, although if you pick and choose they won't hurt you. Produce and dried beans are safe enough anywhere.

Growing sprouts is pretty easy. They are a great source of protein. I myself failed to follow the simple instructions, but perhaps you'll have better luck.

Raising chickens seems to be all the rage. I read a New Yorker article about the particular attraction girls have for the occupation. It teaches responsibility and provides fresh eggs. My co-worker sold eggs on the side, and would notify his customers by raising an egg flag above his cubicle when the crop came in.

Gardens are the best food source of them all. Grow lots. I have a shady lot. The tomatoes would just be getting red when they froze. Basil did best. It goes well in soups, sandwiches, stir-fry, pasta, etc. You just pick what you need fresh off the plant. The inconvenient truth is, your garden will mature at the same time as everybody else's, when there is a fresh food surplus. If you can rotate your crops, so that 1/12 of the harvest comes up each month, let me know how you did it.

CSA shares are a great idea too. I don't do it, because ½ share is too much for me, and I suspect ¼ share would be too. I considered sharing with my neighbor, but wrote it off as too complicated. I try and keep things simple. All else being equal buy local. Why not?

What about Neolithic food that you don't have to pay for? Yes, you can still hunt and gather. This will supplement your larder with natural healthy food. You probably won't come home with a mastodon, but you might collect blackberries, clams, deer, moose, greens, and mushrooms.

So it turns out that there are many places to buy food. If you have not tried all of the aforementioned places, it behooves you to try some of them. If you stick to the All-Food twin pillars, no chemicals and only one ingredient, then food from any of these sources will work well for your body.

FOOD MANAGEMENT, STORAGE AND WASTE

I have always thought that it's wrong to waste food. The Chinese are no longer starving, and it's impractical to fed-ex our leftovers to Somalia, so that leaves us with good food management.

You'll want to stock staples. You'll have pretty rows of glass jars containing rice, beans of various colours, pasta, nuts, spices, flour and other assorted sundries. These don't go bad for a while, and form the foundation of many meals. There will always be something to eat in the house.

Your fridge may not be empty, but it won't be full either. It contains veggies, a little dairy, and a few other things. You don't need that door full of seldom-used things. You don't need dozens of condiments. Keep track of what is in your fridge, and FIFO it before it goes bad. That's computer jargon for First In First Out. That is, try and eat the old stuff before buying too many new perishables. Food containing seafood, meat, and dairy should be eaten relatively quickly. Veggies last longer. Think ahead. If you have too much, trade or gift with your neighbor. My neighbor gets Costco quantities, and gives me a portion, some of which I return in the form of cooked dishes. When leaving home for a weekend or longer, think ahead, consume, don't accumulate. Eat your food, bring it to lunch, give it away. Pursue the goal of zero food waste. Food is a gift from the earth. About half the food produced in America is wasted. Do your part to change this statistic.

RESTAURANTS

Restaurant food won't be as good as your own. It tends to be fatty and costs more too. Cutting down on meals out will help a lot. When you do go out, there are things you can do to minimize the damage to your health.

Portioning is one of the main issues. Restaurants like to overfeed you. You don't want to throw away anything, and it's too much to eat, so the reasonable thing to do it to take it home with you. This works better for certain types of food. With Asian for example, you can order the box right with the meal, as a reminder that your tummy is not the only place to put the food on your table. When you've had enough, and there is a still a pile on the table, box it up and take it home. When you get home, make extra rice if you don't already have some in the fridge. This will stretch out the leftovers, and replaces some fatty food with lean clean rice. You may get days of eating out of a single restaurant meal. This also works for takeout.

Now ask yourself, how often do you order food in a restaurant that you can't finish? I'd wager pretty often. How often do you leave the restaurant unsatisfied, feeling that you under ordered? Virtually never. Keep this in mind, and order less and less. Share more. Split the dish. In the unlikely event that it's insufficient, you can order more. I went to a Tex-Mex place with co-workers, and ordered just a bowl of soup for lunch. It was still too much. They all had extra food to share. No matter how little you order, you will be surprised to find that it may be plenty, or even too much.

In short, plan to eat or take home everything you order

from restaurants.

I keep raving about Asian foods, but some Chinese restaurants are to be avoided. Here are the warning signs:

• Food is sitting in warmers
• The menu includes chop suey and chow mein
• Police officers are eating there
• The restaurant is in a strip mall
• It's a chain

What do you do when faced by unlimited food, as in a buffet or potluck? Here are some strategies. We'd hate to be trim and proper and active all week and then eat ten thousand calories in a sitting. Right off the bat, the sign may say 'all you can eat' but you don't have to eat it all. Have one plate. Stop there, or have a little more. And use smaller plates. What do you put on this plate? Something green, and something unfried. At a potluck you can honor the homemade dishes by sampling them, in lieu of the purchased items. Put good things on your plate and not too many, and this will reduce the damage that an occasional indulgence incurs.

Where do we go for dinner? In the USA, this means "from what country do the recipes come from, not including ours?" My top choices are Asian, oriental, and far eastern. This type of food tends to include healthful grains and vegetables, and ideally is not all fried. The options for protein are tofu, mock duck, seafood, and regular old meat in moderation.

On the other hand, fast food and fried food are to be avoided. Rounding out the rest of the world, Italian food can be heavy. As is French, although the French people eat moderately. Traditional Mexican food is pretty lean, but the Tex-Mex Americanization of it adds calories. If you love any particular cuisine, go ahead and chow down with moderation. Middle eastern food tends to be quite healthy. Nuevo Cousine can offer healthy meals with less fat.

Speaking of dining out, do you like ma and pa places? Sure you do. It's a pity your children won't be able to enjoy them. Every day one of them closes and is replaced by a chain restaurant owned by MomCo and PopCo Inc. Do the math, someday the last one will shut its doors forever. How do we reverse this trend? Avoid chains. Tell your friends and co-workers. When the subject of where to eat comes up, pipe up and state your preference.

Let's say you are meeting a friend, co-worker, or date for dinner. This may lead to high quantities of less than healthful food. To ameliorate the unhealthful effects, meet before dinner for a stroll at a nearby park. Equally effective is a digestive stroll afterward.

MEAT

Let talk about meat.

The most important thing is that the meat you eat has eaten real food. One of the main reasons to avoid meat is factory farms. They pollute and use lots of water. What's worse, the animals are given antibiotics, growth hormones, and who knows what else. So if you do eat meat, which is OK in moderation, try and avoid factory farms.

In terms of your health, vegetarianism is optional. This was once a polarizing issue. Remember when the hitchhiker said "What! You allow the flesh of murdered animals to enter the holy temple of your body?" Things have changed. You don't have to go veggie, but if you do, you will lose more weight. I was a pescatarian (fish eater) for a while, which also works. If you go vegan, you will be hard pressed to gain an ounce. In this case, be very careful to get enough protein and vitamins.

Also note that avoiding meat means eating lower on the food chain. This has several benefits. No one ever got Mad Tofu Disease, because farmers don't grind up tofu brains and feed them to young tofettes. It also conserves the world's food supply. My second stint as a veggie was in part fueled by the statistic that it takes ten pounds of grain to make a pound of meat. In addition to grain, the modern method of raising animals in feedlots uses more fertilizer, pesticides, antibiotics, growth hormones, oil, and water. If everyone ate more grain, fed less to cattle, and ate less meat, we'll all be a bit healthier, and there would be more food in the world. Would everyone then get enough to eat? Not necessarily. There would still be uneven distribution. But the karmic balance of the earth would improve.

On the other hand, suppose you let animals graze, roam the range, and eat their natural diet. This avoids most of the aforementioned issues. Cows like to eat grass. They are built for it. Animals like to range free. It makes then happy. What makes cows really unhappy? Grazing on AstroTurf. Lets hope it never comes to this.

Grains are good, and animals are good too, as long as they weren't raised on a factory farm, they ate natural food, and they weren't given chemicals. In fact, you could say that animals too need to follow the All-Food Diet. This makes them healthy, and the benefit is passed on to you when you eat them.

GO AHEAD AND HAVE THESE ONCE A YEAR

Soda is OK once a year. Americans drink on average 600 sodas a year. They get 10% of their calories from soda. I set of a goal of having one a year. Occasionally I feel the need for a stomach-soothing ginger ale on a plane. Every year I have more than one, but that's OK. If you do have an occasional soda, try to choose a natural one without corn syrup.

There are only three things wrong with soda. Caffeine, high fructose corn syrup, artificial sweeteners, and chemicals. What amazes me is that I see people giving soda, even caffeinated soda, to their small children. Children should drink milk, water, and juice. Even one soda a year may be too many for them.

Donuts aren't exactly health food either. Again, I aim for one per year, and if I go over a bit, I'm still doing OK. If there is a choice at work, consider selecting a scone or bagel.

PREPARED FOODS AND PICNICS

Prepared foods that are ready to eat from supermarkets are becoming increasingly popular. This is the worst of both worlds. The unhealthiness and expense of restaurant food, without the ambiance. Try to avoid them. You are better off cooking for yourself most of the time, and going out for something healthy the rest of the time.

Whatever you eat, cooking at home will usually be cheaper, healthier, and lower in calories than going out. So walk to the grocery store and the farmers market, buy some real food, and cook it. Invite your friends. You don't have to cook every day. You can cook up a large dish on Sunday, and break it into small lunch and dinner portions. You can freeze some of them. If you have time after work, turn on the radio and cook, even if you are not hungry. The food will be there when you need it, helping you resist the temptation to spend money.

Are all your meals based on Meat & Potatoes? The all American diet is not so great. If you were weaned on it, you'll have to work at changing how you think about dinner. Meals don't need to be centered on these foods. Stir-fry, casseroles, and soups can make a meal. These contain lots of rice, beans, and vegetables, and smaller quantities of dairy and meat.

Fried food is to be avoided. Look out for restaurants where everything is fried. Occasionally, it's OK. If it's a regular thing with you, start thinking about alternatives.

Sometimes I find myself at an all American scary picnic. I ask myself, what is food? What is real food? While my diet seems natural to me, others find their own diets to be natural to them. They grew up eating canned, fatty, artificial food. I find these picnic food selections horrifying. It's all meat, fat, sugar, white bread, and canned fruit and other non-food items. In this situation, one has to make the best of it, be polite, and keep an eye out for real food somewhere in the mix.

Frozen food is better than canned. I avoid it as well though, because it's not fresh. What should there be in your freezer? Not much. Just ice, ice cream, and small portions of the large batches of soup and stew that you made. Freezing the food you cook is OK, as is canning the food you grow.

Do you know how to potluck? It's a great way to be social without spending a lot. It's easy. Bring something. Cook it yourself, deli food is lame. Your goal should be not to scrape by, but to bring the loveliest dish. Bringing a veggie dish is more inclusive. Casseroles are a big hit. Soups invoke the three hand issue. One for your plate, one for the bowl, one to serve yourself with. This is why I don't bring soups anymore. The bottom line is, if you made it yourself, you've done well. I find it difficult to eat moderately. If someone goes to the trouble of making food, I find it disrespectful not to sample it. Sometimes I find that I've already pre-eaten the next meal. Yes, it appears that I've told you to eat three meals a day and also to skip meals. Eat three meals, unless there are extenuating circumstances, such as lateness of the hour, or having indulged in a supersized buffet or potluck. Then you can skip a meal.

KITCHEN GEAR

Microwaves are not good. I came to my senses, and sold mine on Craigslist. I got $20 for it, and it freed up some valuable kitchen space. I hated the beeps and the way it heated unevenly, with some parts of the food burning hot and other parts ice cold. While there is nothing unhealthy about them, they have no useful function in the home. You can heat up food and water on the stove, the way our foremothers did. The only thing I miss is the clock. Someday, I'll find a cute analog clock at a garage sale and enshrine it in my little kitchen.

Teflon is the devil's material. Someday they'll decide whether or not it causes Alzheimer's. I'm not waiting around to find out. And the way it flakes off? Where do the flakes go? Into your dinner. And who is meticulous about not using metal implements with them? Lose the Teflon now. The best places to put Teflon pans are thrift stores and the garbage bin.

Cast iron is great. The frying pans last forever, and you get a bit of iron in your diet. Get a few of them. I also have a dutch oven with legs for putting into campfires. It has a heavy lid to keep out ash and sand. Revere Ware is nice too. And of course there is that mainstay, the wok.

And a word about how to use a stove. First light the burner. Then turn down the flame, so that it doesn't escape out around the edge of the pan, melting the handle, wasting energy, and making the pan too hot to pick up. Heating the handle and sides of the pan does not make water boil any faster. When cooking rice, simmering food, cooking with milk, or reheating leftovers, use the lowest possible heat setting and be patient. Add a little water if needed. The food will cook and heat evenly and will not burn.

Bread machines sure are easy. For sure, it's better to make bread by hand. Mea culpa. Except for carrot bread and banana bread, I use the machine because it's so much easier. Unfortunately the texture is inferior, and the bread tends to be too soft. I use a whole-wheat setting, with the darkest crust setting, and let it sit a few hours when it's done to ensure further hardening.

Either way, making your own bread lets you know what's in it, and what's not in it. Whole wheat is better. If the recipe calls for white, try half and half. You can try all whole wheat, but it may not work. Bread making is after all a matter of chemistry. If you do experiment, alter just one thing at a time. This may prevent catastrophic recipe failure.

Now that I've dispensed so much advice, I feel motivated to bake bread. Stay tuned for the second edition and see if I follow through. Late note: Nope, not baking yet.

I miss my teakettle. It tooted its last whistle and bit the dust with a leak. They do a fine job of heating water. The whistle will help you to not burn all your pans the way I do. Update: I found another on eBay.

Plastic isn't great stuff. I try and avoid it. I store dry food in glass jars. My implements are wood, metal, or glass. If you are lacking some items, try garage sales. Flippers, measuring cups, measuring spoons, and other kitchen items should not be made of plastic.

I like my rice cooker. It's handy that it keeps rice warm, and doesn't burn it. The instruction book says to use less water. Ignore this. First wash the rice. For each cup of rice, add two cups water for white rice, two and a half cups for brown rice. Brown rice has more nutritive value. If you prefer white, feel free, but try and make brown more often. Rice is a staple. I keep mine in a big glass jar. But don't get too much, and be careful of bulk rice, lest you find bugs in it.

I shouldn't have to mention this, but a TV is one of those appliances that doesn't belong in the kitchen. And if there is one there, it should not be on during meals. Or at any other time.

Cookbooks are useful for making real food. Everyone should own *Laurel's Kitchen*. I buy piles of them at Overstock.com, and give them away for weddings and other occasions. I also like Deborah Madison's *Vegetarian Cooking for Everyone*. Mollie Katzen's *Moosewood Cookbook* is good one, although some of the recipes are a tad complex. *The Joy of Cooking* covers a lot, just temper it with a bias towards fresh produce and whole grains. Try to avoid too many cookbooks that call for unhealthy food, canned food, non-whole foods, and the like. There are also a zillion recipes online.

That was a lot of advice on food. Lets sum it up: Buy foods with one ingredient. Avoid canned, processed, and frozen food. Cook. Shop in the right place.

ACTIVE LIFESTYLE

I could tell you to exercise, and I probably will. But you knew that. More helpful are suggestions on simple day-to-day things, like parking and using stairs. Being active should be part of your regular day. Let's talk about both now, starting with being active. It's not necessarily an exercise program, it's just part of your day.

Walking is the easiest way to be active. Just walk. Walk to the store. Stroll for pleasure. Take a digestive stroll.

When you drive and are near your destination, park in the first spot you see. You'll save a few seconds and a teaspoon of gas, and you'll be on your feet where you belong. In hard to park areas, park blocks away, on residential streets. Don't pay to park, but be early and willing to walk a spell. This may not work in New York City. On the other hand, it worked well in San Francisco. You can find free parking by heading away from shops and towards residential streets. Then you walk back to your destination.

Another variation of this theme applies when you have several stops to make in your car. Drive to the 'main destination', be it the nearest or the one where you are buying the heaviest stuff, and walk back and forth and across the street to the others. This small change of habits will again save you a teaspoon of gas and add a little more 'activeness' to your lifestyle.

Being active every day is what we are focusing on. This is a key point. You can incorporate being active into your lifestyle. You do this by walking and biking places such as work, the market, and social activities. Or you can do some honest manual labour. One day this month I biked to a friends house, push-mowed his lawn, and biked home. I could have driven, but chose not to. Another day I biked to a friend's house and tore all the shingles off his roof. This ate up most of the days, but the weather was nice, I had little else to do, and it seemed like a win-win situation to get exercise and make a few bucks at the same time.

"Blow up your TV, throw away your papers, move to the country". These John Prine lyrics contain some food for thought. Lots of people claim that they "don't watch TV", but somehow watch more than they intend. How can we rectify this? The first step is to lose cable. It's a waste of money and nothing is ever on, even with a thousand channels. If you can go whole hog, lose the TV, especially if you have kids. Everyone will spend more time outdoors, and interact more creatively. This may lead to spending time talking, singing, and playing. This is what previous generations did. Who would of thought that would ever happen again?

Can you throw away your papers? This isn't terribly practical today. What you can do is to do business with as few companies as possible. This generates less paper and stress. Simplify. An ex was stressed about her checking account, and bouncing checks. I advised her to close the account, and buy money orders to pay bills. Back then, this worked well.

Move to the country? A fine idea. It's cheap, and with UPS and the Internet, more people can get by living away from urban areas. When you get there, don't forget to walk and bike everywhere.

Another way to be more active is to get a dog. Your dog needs to be walked. You do too, but you may not know it. Fido can be your excuse to increase your activity and health.

Do you work in an office? Here is an easy one. Step out once a day and circumnavigate the building. Do you have a harmonica, or a penny-whistle? Take them with you, and let loose for five minutes a day. Over time your playing will improve. Now that I think about it, you could read as well. Find some green space near work, and walk there. Read for a few minutes, and walk back.

I've worked downtown, and in Northern, Southern, Eastern, and Western suburbs. My friends live all over town. The one constant is my desire to go to the Y every day. Note that I said desire. I don't actually make it every day.

What did I do? I moved really close to my Y. It's so close, that I can pop in for short sessions, even when I lack motivation to do a full workout. Now I'm not asking you to move today, but if you happen to be moving, which many of us do all too often, look for a place near the gym and other amenities that you can walk or bike to.

TWO WHEELS GOOD, FOUR WHEELS BAD

Biking is a key part of the All-Food Diet. Hopefully you live somewhere amenable to biking. There are several factors that could make it hard to bike. Bad weather is one. While there are year round bikers in the Twin Cities, I give it up when it's rainy, icy, quite windy, or below 20 degrees. Above that temperature in sunny weather biking is quite feasible given a few layers and gloves. Another obstacle is traffic. Bike paths are rare enough. Bike lanes can be useful, provided that they are not just road-paint. If there are side roads, they will have less traffic. Lastly, distance can be an issue. If you live miles from nowhere, you have a few options. You can get yourself into supershape, bike one way, or get a battery assist bike. For some people none of the above will be practical. Do the best you can.

Where can you bike to? Everywhere of course, but particularly to buy food. This is after all a diet book. Too much to carry? Take your kids and put backpacks on them. Put a carry sack on your dog. Pull your little red wagon. Be creative.

One of the difficulties of walking and biking to buy food is the weight, especially with liquids. So when you do drive, buy a few months worth of sparkling water and juice. Beer and wine present another issue. Will your roommates consume it all the day that you buy it? Will you? If the answer to these two questions is an unequivocal "no", then go ahead and stock up. You'll save some gas, and when you walk or bike to buy provisions, you'll only need to buy non-liquids or perishables, and they won't weigh as much.

When I was working in Baton Rouge, it was hard to bike to work. For one thing, it was saunific. Even early morning was hot. I had a co-worker from New York, who didn't own a car. His solution was a power assist bike, with a battery pack. He'd ride to work for pennies and arrived in a sweat-free condition.

Cars are bad, for numerous reasons. Can you live without one? Many people used to. Not coincidentally, people used to be more fit as well. Can your household get by with one less car? Or can you park yours, and take it out for exercise on Sunday? That's what I aim for.

How do you get here and there without a car? By bus, trolley, horse, subway, train, walking, or biking. Did I mention pogo stick? Share a ride with a friend. Accept one way rides. Someone at the event will take you home, or you can walk. You'll get home somehow, never fear.

Let's say the post office is a mile away. You need to go there, but you don't get around it to. It's an errand that is stuck on your todo list, and it is increasing your stress level. One fine Saturday you treat yourself to a leisurely stroll. You do the errand and feel good about it.

Bike riding is a multi-win situation. It's good exercise, saves on gas and wear and tear on your car, gets you outdoors, can be social, and gives you an excuse to go places.

You'll want to carry lots of food and other items on your bike. I use a rack and saddlebags, square ones that are shaped like grocery bags. In fact, the grocery bags rise above the saddlebags to carry even more. I've seen bikes hauling coolers and other large containers. You can also drop food into those child haulers.

While everyone should have a bike, they should not have your bike. I had three bikes stolen one year. None of them had a U-shaped lock. I hear about stolen bikes all the time. The one common theme? They didn't have U-shaped locks. Get a U-shaped lock. I have several now, and my bikes no longer run away. If I tie up in a questionable location, I use an additional cable to secure the wheels.

Here is an easy one. Walk to get your mail. Some people drive amazingly short distances to get mail.

Do you live in a multi-person household? If you have partner or child who isn't working too much, they can help the whole house live a healthier lifestyle. Yes, child labour has its place. Pry them away from the screen, and share the kitchen with them. Teenagers are fully capable of cooking an entire meal. Pre-teens can assist with many chores, albeit sharp things and hot things are unsuitable for certain ages. Buying, growing, and preparing your own food is a way of turning spare time into savings and health. Those with spare time can take advantage of this. Those that do go to work will leave the house with their lunchboxes full.

PLAIN OLD ORDINARY EXERCISE

Actual exercise, as opposed to active lifestyle, can be done solo or with others. Both have their advantages, and really it's a matter of personal choice. Some people are more motivated to exercise when they are part of a crowd. They do well in a class setting, where someone tells them what to do and everyone else is doing it. Others prefer to be active by themselves. They run, climb mountains, ski, whatever. Is that you? Good, go with it. At a loss? Here are some ways to exercise.

Tai chi isn't particularly strenuous, and helps balance, focus, muscle tone, and overall karma. I had eventually learned 108 movements before forgetting them again. Any other martial art has the same benefits. The styles range from soft to hard, with tai chi being on the soft end. The hard end has more to do with combat and kicking people in the head. As I said, all have their benefits, but I noticed that devotees over time gravitate to the softer arts, which have more in common with dance than fighting.

Yoga has similar benefits, and is enormously popular nowadays. Everyone and their sister is doing yoga. It's good for you. I'm partial to Kundalini, but any style will do you good.

This is a good time to mention dancing. Many improbably out of shape people can move to the music. If you don't dance, try a class. It will be more fun than basic training.

Wake up. Most of us do this in the morning. Do you own a floor? I suspected as much. Lie on it and do your favorite mini-set. Every day. Mini-sets are short exercise routines. Mine is 108 ab crunches, 30 leg lifts right left and on tummy, some pushups, cat-cows, an occasional cat stretch, and maybe a yoga tree. The routine varies, and sometimes I slack off. The basics take about five minutes. Most everyone can spare that much time. Is this a complete workout? No. Are there a hundred million Americans that get less exercise than this? Yes. If you have a mat and a bar, you can use them as well. If you feel like doing a full set, be it 30, 60, or 90 minutes, go ahead, make me feel like a wimp.

Running is simplicity itself, involving little equipment. You can run alone or with others. But you say, my running partner talks too much, goes too slow, stops too often. What can you do? You find a circular route, be it a lake, a park or a trail. Then you head off in opposite directions. When you meet in the middle, you have two choices. You can wave and keep going until you both reach the starting point. Or if you've both had enough, you can stroll back together.

Zumba in my favorite class. It involves lots of motion, Latin music, and dance moves. My teacher is from Brazil, as are some of the students. There is also a good sized Somali contingent. It seems to have universal appeal.

Some of you are large. Some of you have knee and joint problems. Some of you are unwieldy or otherwise ill suited to walking or biking. Here is where swimming comes in. It can be laps, treading water, aqua classes, or just moseying around. It's hard to hurt anything, and you'll be getting in shape. Even if it's just five minutes, cool off and splash a bit. If you are near coral and fish, grab a snorkel, it's pretty neat.

See those runners and skiers in ankle casts and crutches? None of them were swimming when it happened. Soaking in the hot tub is pleasant, but does not qualify as exercise. However, you can swim as few as three laps and call it part of an active day. If you are a fish, and swim miles, you've got me beat.

I'm fond of the Nordic Trak. They are easy on the knees, and readily available. My first one I bought used for $300. I had stored it at a girlfriend's house, and she said she tossed it during a cleaning. Looking in the basement, I saw the 'thrown away' object, sans skis. She had no idea where the skis were. Later on I saw a nice looking Nordic Trak for sale on the side of the road. I tried to buy the skis, but they didn't want a skiless machine, and so for $50 I ended up owning a second Nordic Trak. Later still, we tried to make skis out of wood. It's easy enough, but we failed with the bindings. So, a few years later, I'm biking to work through an alley, and I see some Nordic Trak skis by a dumpster. It's at an exercise equipment shop, and I pop in the garage and ask the guys if I can have the skis. I stick them in my bike bag (they poke up about 6 feet out of it), and carefully ride to work. A few years later, I'm taking a walk and looking for garage sales. I see a Nordic Trak on the side of the road with a free sign, and it's mine. So now I own three Nordic Traks. Make me an offer, and I'll give you two for the price of one.

Playing with children is a good way to wear yourself out. Adults can be boring, they just sit around talk. When I'm in an all ages social group, my first thought is to play with the junior set. While drawing and chess aren't really active, the Aerobie has been a big hit. It flies like a Frisbee, but goes twice as far. To catch it, raise your arm, and the ring will fall over it like magic.

THINGS TO AVOID

Elevators. Just say no. Here are some reasons:

• Walking stairs is good exercise. While you are at it, use the stairs to do some calf lifts every day. If it's too many stairs to walk up, just walk down.

• Avoid that awkward time, too short to converse, long enough to be uncomfortable as you both stare at the floor number display.

• Save energy.

• Sooner or later, it's going to get stuck and you won't be on it. Yay.

• It's unlikely that the elevator will free fall, but it is even more unlikely that the stairs you are walking on will collapse.

• It can save your life. I had a co-worker who was in good shape. He had a large brood of children and a boyish aspect to him. He liked stairs. On 9/11 he was working in the World Trade Center, and he walked down 40 flights of stairs and out the door, safe and sound.

Power mowers are evil. Why use a push mower?

- You get exercise
- They take fewer resources to manufacture
- They don't drink oil and gas
- They need fewer repairs
- They last longer
- They are easier to dispose of
- They are blessedly quieter

If it's a large yard, do a little at a time. Yes I know, if you have 40 acres this will just not work for most people. That's OK, you thought about it.

This applies to snow blowers too. If the snow is heavy, put a few flakes at a time on your shovel, it'll be easier on the back.

Speaking of backs, many people have back trouble. Mine got better after I settled on this regimen:

- Get the firmest possible mattress. When visiting places with soft beds, sleep on the floor, which can be padded with a few blankets.

- Do ab crunches every day.

- Sit up straight, no slouching.

- Raise your PC monitor with some phone books, reams of paper, or a milk crate, so that it's significantly higher than your keyboard. Your eyes are in your head, which is easily a foot above desk level.

- Use a wrist rest for both keyboard and mouse.

- Adjust the car seat so that you sit straighter.

Bags are to be avoided. Since you buy real food, it will come with less disposable packaging. Voila, you don't need garbage bags. I never understood the need for them. You throw away paper and plastic bags, and buy other bags? This is an easy way to be green. Put your trash in your shopping bags. You'll probably still have too many bags, so bring cloth bags to the market sometimes and it will all balance out.

Smoking is the baddest of the bad. You can eat right and have an active lifestyle, but you aren't healthy if you smoke. Your corpse may be trim, but your friends will miss you. When you light up, you are sending out a message that reads "I don't care to see my grandchildren grow up". Besides, cigarettes have zillions of ingredients. No, you can't have natural tobacco either.

Just say no to Walmart on general principles. Make it a point not to set foot in it. This will help make the world a better place. I also avoid the golden arches, the archetype of unhealthy eating.

You may also find that you don't need a dishwasher. If you don't have one, yay, don't get one. If it breaks, you don't have to replace it. If you already have one, well, that's your call. Dishwashers use energy, are noisy, and you have to prewash the dishes. Hand washing dishes is a Zen activity, a social activity, a time to listen to the radio and work with your hands in the warm water.

Dryers use energy and hurt your clothes. Hang them up, and they will last longer and smell better. If it's damp and cold, hang them indoors. It may take a few days, but they will dry eventually. And guess what? You don't really need fabric softener, it's just something the corporations invented to take more of your money.

OTHER WAYS TO BE GREEN

Eating at work, at a market, at a deli, or at someone else's house can produce lots of waste. This is easy to avoid. You can keep a coffee cup at work for drinks and water, and a plate and a bowl, and some silverware. You can carry some silverware or reusable plasticware in your glove box and in your bike basket. You can carry hankies or dishcloths for cleanups in place of paper. Styrofoam is the worst offender, but it's good for momma earth to use less plastic and paper as well. Sometimes when I'm at a party or potluck I'll run out to the van to get my own cup or utensil. Other times I'll just raid the host's cupboard for a real fork.

What about being green on the green? Is golf ecologically friendly? My old German roomie was confounded by these sorts of questions. "How does eating tuna kill golfers?" he asked us. I would have to encourage you to walk nine rather than drive eighteen. My neighbor once built a 3-hold course on the beach, which got good use by the retirees. Walking is good.

Now that I think about it, there are other sources of chemicals in our lives besides food. There are cleaners, disinfectants, insecticides, and the like. Are there replacements for these with one natural ingredient? Perhaps not. Many of these products are not strictly necessary, having been invented in recent generations by corporations and touted by Madison Avenue. Others can be used sparingly in special circumstances. A good rule of thumb is to buy as few chemicals as possible. The poisons inevitable get into the air, water, and your skin and lungs, and one can't think that they are in any way beneficial.

WHAT WOULD JESUS EAT

What Would Jesus Eat? How did Jesus live? Did he live his life in accordance with these ideas? Well, I'm pretty certain he didn't drive a car, or even ride a bicycle. He walked everywhere, getting plenty of exercise. He ate simple chemical free foods, and adhered to a Mediterranean diet. He ate meat sparingly, and drank wine, but not to excess. He ate fish and whole grain bread. He shared food, and certainly didn't waste any. He didn't use disposable dishes. He didn't eat fast food, canned food, frozen food, or processed food. He had an active lifestyle and ate simple food.

Does all this seem like a lot to remember? Let's sum it up again: Walk, ride, play, and buy foods with only one ingredient.

THE ALL-FOOD DIET ONLINE.

Please visit the blog and FaceBook page. Feel free to ask any questions, post any thoughts or ideas you may have, or just talk about your health, the things you did (or didn't) do today, food, activity, or whatever interests you.

www.facebook.com/AllFoodDiet

AllFoodDiet.blogspot.com

www.amzn.com/gp/product/148009966X

www.goodreads.com/book/show/16145627-the-all-food-diet

RECIPES

Pho

Prep/cooking time: 20 minutes

Fill large Pot with water about 2/3 full
Set burner on Hi
Slice veggies to desired size
Stir sporadically as you add ingredients

Add:
Serrano or Jalapeno pepper
Bundle of sliced green onions

Turn down heat to low and add:
Miso or other veggie soup stock base (use sparingly)
Hot Sesame oil (or other oil), many drops
Lime. Squeeze lots of lime in till stock tastes sour
Pepper, to taste
Lots of soy sauce or tamari, to taste

After veggies are cooked, add:
Package of hard (or firm) tofu
One Roma tomato
Package of rice noodles

Rice noodles will be cooked in about three minutes
Serve when they are soft

Serve with basil and sprouts

Curry Rice

Fry a green onion in hot oil

Optionally, Add:
Bits of sliced veggies, such as cabbage or bok choy
Tofu
Peanuts

Add:

Rice

Curry Paste (there must be a way to make your own, can someone post it)

Sliced Roma Tomato

Cubed jack cheese (optional)

Cook till hot and serve

Mexican V8 soup

In a medium saucepan, put 1 to 2 cans of Jugo de Verduras Ocho. In a pinch, substitute American V8. Fill pan with water till it's ½ full. Put on High.

Add:

Pepper
Hot Pepper oil (a few drops)
2 Sliced Anaheim chilis
Several green onions and/or regular onion
Lots of cabbage
Lots of potatoes
Other veggies as desired

Serve with bread

Salad and Potatoes

Left side of plate:

Pour some peanut sauce on romaine lettuce

Right side of plate:

Slice some unpeeled potatoes real small

Boil till soft

Serve with butter and soy sauce or tamari

Note: Peanut sauce can be made from peanuts, coconut milk, spices and a few other things. I've never done it though.

Pasta with veggie garnish

Use small quantities of everything

Cook in hot oil:

Green onions
Roma tomato
Cabbage

Optional ingredients

Broccoli
Black Olives
Brussel Sprouts

Put on top of pasta

Yuppie pasta or angel hair work well

Tacos Veracruzana

Protein can be eggs, fish, or shrimp among other thing

Or you can use cabbage instead

Fry in hot oil:

One Jalapeno or Serrano pepper

Anaheim pepper (optional)

Add Onion

Red pepper (optional)

Wait

Add lime & romas

Add protein

Heat tortillas on top, one by one

Coconut Curry

Canola Oil
Curry
Onion
Anaheim pepper
Cashews, Almond slivers, sunflower seeds
Pea Pods
Red Pepper
Corn (cut from cob)
Coconut milk
Curry paste
Pepper
Hot sauce
Soy sauce or tamari

Add and stir fry in order given

Serve with rice

Fish Chowder

Cook an onion in oil

Add potatoes

Cook a bit longer

Add milk

Add cut up Tilapia

Add salt, pepper, and cumin or curry powder

FACTS AND FIGURES

Americans drink on average 600 sodas a year

http://www.everyday-wisdom.com/soft-drink-consumption.html

They get 10% of their calories from soda

http://articles.cnn.com/2007-09-18/health/kd.liquid.calories_1_nondiet-drinks-hfcs-soda?_s=PM:HEALTH

About half the food produced in America is wasted.

http://www.foodproductiondaily.com/Supply-Chain/Half-of-US-food-goes-to-waste

http://www.culinate.com/articles/features/wasted_food

BIBLIOGRAPHY

Cranz, Galen. The Chair: Rethinking Culture, Body, and Design.

Katzen, Mollie. The Moosewood Cookbook.

Madison, Deborah. Vegetarian Cooking for Everyone.

Pollan, Michael. In Defense of Food.

Pollan, Michael. The Omnivore's Dilemma.

Robertson, Laurel. Laurels Kitchen.

Wasserman, Debra. Simply Vegan.

ABOUT THE AUTHOR

Hans Guttmann is a computer programmer.

In his real life, he reads, cooks, bikes, sings, strums, and camps on the beach in Mexico in his VW poptop.

He currently resides in Minneapolis.

He can be reached at <u>hansguttmann@gmail.com</u>

Made in the USA
San Bernardino, CA
12 May 2014